COOKBOOK DIABETES GUIDE FOR ZERO SUGAR

Zero Sugar, Full Flavor: The Ultimate Diabetes Cookbook

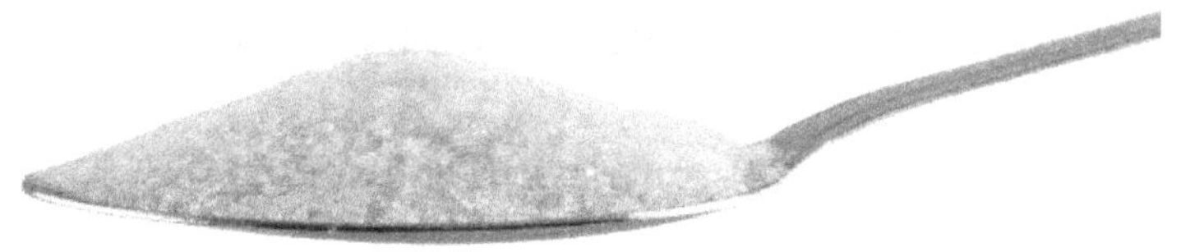

Bernard D. Nelson

INTRODUCTION

Jenny became embroiled in the complications of managing her diabetes in the fast-paced world of today's society. Her continual juggling of work, family, and health had left her longing for a lifeline that would enable her to turn her challenges into victories on a regular basis. During this difficult time, she discovered a book that would become a literary ally and a ray of hope: the "Cookbook Diabetes Guide for Zero Sugar."

Looking through the pages of this cookbook, Jenny found more than recipes; she found a guide to a life free from the chains of too much sugar. The book turned into a silent companion, taking her on a culinary adventure that not only piqued her interest but also fed her body in ways she never would have imagined.

From sweet treats to savory treats, every recipe in the "Cookbook Diabetes Guide for Zero Sugar" served as a springboard for Jenny's journey toward a better way of living. Jenny noticed a significant improvement in her health as she ate the thoughtfully chosen meals and realized the life-changing potential of mindful eating and low-sugar living.

Come along as we unravel Jenny's inspirational story through the pages of a cookbook that served as her ally, mentor, and, in the end, the spark that propelled her on her victorious road toward a life with diabetes that is not a barrier but rather a chapter filled with delicious possibilities and power.

When it comes to cooking and living a healthy lifestyle, the "Cookbook Diabetes Guide for Zero Sugar" is a flavorful and empowering resource. A revolution in taste as well as in the fundamentals of how we view and treat diabetes is revealed in the pages of this culinary manual. This cookbook is a full voyage into a world where delicious dishes harmonize with the ideals of zero-sugar living, as the title suggests. It's beyond a compilation of recipes.

This cookbook is irresistible not just because of its delicious dishes but also because of its ability to completely change the lives of people managing diabetes. It's a well-put-together collection that goes above and beyond the norm, providing a wide range of tasty treats without sacrificing health. Readers will go on a culinary journey via these pages, learning how to prepare meals that satisfy the palate while also adhering to the stringent requirements of a zero-sugar diet.

Come explore the mysteries of this gastronomic treasure trove with us, where every recipe represents a step toward a happier, healthier life. This cookbook is more than simply a reference; it's a traveling companion that will help us rethink the connection between diabetes and the pleasure of food. Allow the "Cookbook Diabetes Guide for Zero Sugar" to serve as your ticket to a world where health and flavor collide, transforming every meal into a celebration of life

Chapter 1

Getting Started with a Zero Sugar Diet

Embarking on the journey of a zero sugar diet marks a pivotal step towards proactive health management, especially for individuals dealing with diabetes. This chapter serves as your compass, navigating through the foundational aspects of initiating and embracing a lifestyle centered around the principles of zero sugar.

1.1 What is a Zero Sugar Diet?

A zero sugar diet is a deliberate dietary approach focused on minimizing or entirely eliminating added sugars from daily nutrition. This lifestyle shift involves a conscious selection of whole, unprocessed foods while avoiding sugary snacks, processed meals, and sweetened beverages. By reducing sugar intake, individuals aim to stabilize blood sugar levels, reduce inflammation, and enhance metabolic health.

Throughout this section, we'll explore the philosophy behind a zero sugar diet, introducing a spectrum of nutritious and satisfying foods that form the core of this approach, fostering a shift towards a more mindful and health-centric relationship with food.

1.2 Benefits for Diabetics

Understanding the profound advantages a zero sugar diet offers to individuals managing diabetes is pivotal. Beyond the direct impact on blood sugar control, this dietary shift contributes significantly to weight management, improved insulin sensitivity, and a decreased risk of diabetes-related complications. Through this segment, we'll delve into the scientific rationale behind these benefits, illustrating how embracing a zero sugar lifestyle can become a cornerstone for enhanced diabetes care and overall well-being.

1.3 Key Principles and Guidelines

Navigating the terrain of a zero sugar diet necessitates understanding and adopting fundamental principles and practical guidelines. This segment equips you with the knowledge needed to seamlessly integrate a sugar-conscious approach into your daily life. From deciphering food labels to making informed choices in various culinary settings, you'll gain insights into the fundamental principles guiding successful adherence to a zero sugar lifestyle.

This chapter acts as your gateway into the empowering realm of a zero sugar diet. By grasping its definition, understanding its profound benefits for individuals managing diabetes, and embracing the key principles and guidelines, you lay the groundwork for a transformative journey towards a healthier, more vibrant you. Welcome to the commencement of change, where every decision made and every meal chosen propels you towards a life defined by mindful, sugar-conscious living.

Chapter 2:

Essential Ingredients for Zero Sugar

Cooking

In the quest for mastering the art of zero sugar cooking, understanding the essential ingredients becomes paramount. This chapter serves as your culinary guide, unveiling a palette of ingredients that not only align with the principles of a zero sugar diet but also contribute to flavorful and nutritious meals.

2.1 Sugar Alternatives

Navigating a zero sugar cooking journey requires reimagining the role of sweetness in recipes. This section explores a spectrum of sugar alternatives that serve as wholesome substitutes. From natural sweeteners like stevia, erythritol, and monk fruit to innovative solutions like date paste and applesauce, you'll discover how these alternatives bring sweetness without the glycemic impact of traditional sugars. We'll delve into their flavor profiles, application methods, and how to seamlessly incorporate them into your favorite recipes.

2.2 Low-Glycemic Index Foods

Understanding the glycemic index is key to managing blood sugar levels effectively. In this section, we'll explore a variety of low-glycemic index foods that not only provide sustained energy but also contribute to the overall health of individuals following a zero sugar cooking approach. Whole grains, legumes, and certain fruits and vegetables become staples in this culinary journey, offering a balance between nutritional richness and glycemic control.

2.3 Healthy Fats and Proteins

Fats and proteins play a crucial role in crafting satisfying and nutritious zero sugar meals. This segment dives into the world of healthy fats, such as avocados, olive oil, and nuts, which contribute richness and flavor to dishes. Additionally, we'll explore lean proteins like poultry, fish, and plant-based sources, highlighting their role in stabilizing blood sugar levels and promoting satiety. Understanding the synergy between fats, proteins, and carbohydrates becomes essential in creating well-rounded, zero sugar recipes.

Throughout this chapter, you'll gain insights into the nuanced world of ingredients that redefine the boundaries of zero sugar cooking. By incorporating sugar alternatives, embracing low-glycemic index foods, and understanding the role of healthy fats and proteins, you'll not only satisfy your palate but also embark on a culinary journey that aligns seamlessly with the principles of a zero sugar lifestyle. Welcome to the heart of the kitchen, where these essential ingredients become the building blocks of delicious, health-conscious meals.

Chapter 3:

Breakfast Delights

As the sun rises on a new day, the journey into the realm of zero sugar cooking unfolds with a focus on the most important meal: breakfast. Chapter 3 explores a delightful array of morning creations that not only tantalize the taste buds but also align with the principles of a zero sugar diet.

3.1 Zero Sugar Smoothies

Start your day on a refreshing note with zero sugar smoothies that burst with natural flavors and wholesome ingredients. This section introduces a variety of vibrant smoothie recipes crafted from a foundation of sugar alternatives like stevia or monk fruit. Packed with nutrient-rich fruits, leafy greens, and protein sources such as Greek yogurt or plant-based protein powder, these smoothies offer a delightful and energizing way to kickstart your morning.

3.2 Nutty Granola Bowl

Indulge in the satisfying crunch of a nutty granola bowl without the added sugars that often accompany store-bought varieties. This part of the chapter explores the art of crafting your granola using a mix of nuts, seeds, and sugar alternatives. Paired with Greek yogurt or a dairy-free alternative and adorned with fresh berries or sliced fruits, this granola bowl becomes a wholesome and filling breakfast option, providing sustained energy throughout the morning.

3.3 Veggie Omelette Surprise

Elevate your breakfast experience with the Veggie Omelette Surprise, a savory and satisfying option that combines the goodness of eggs with a colorful array of vegetables. This section guides you through the art of creating a fluffy omelette without the need for added sugars. From bell peppers and spinach to tomatoes and mushrooms, the Veggie Omelette Surprise not only delights the palate but also ensures a nutrient-packed start to your day.

Throughout Chapter 3, you'll discover that a zero sugar breakfast can be both indulgent and nutritious. By exploring the world of zero sugar smoothies, crafting your nutty granola bowl, and mastering the art of a veggie omelette, you'll embrace breakfast delights that not only satisfy your morning cravings but also set the tone for a day filled with delicious and health-conscious choices. Welcome to the joy of zero sugar breakfasts, where every bite is a celebration of flavor and well-being.

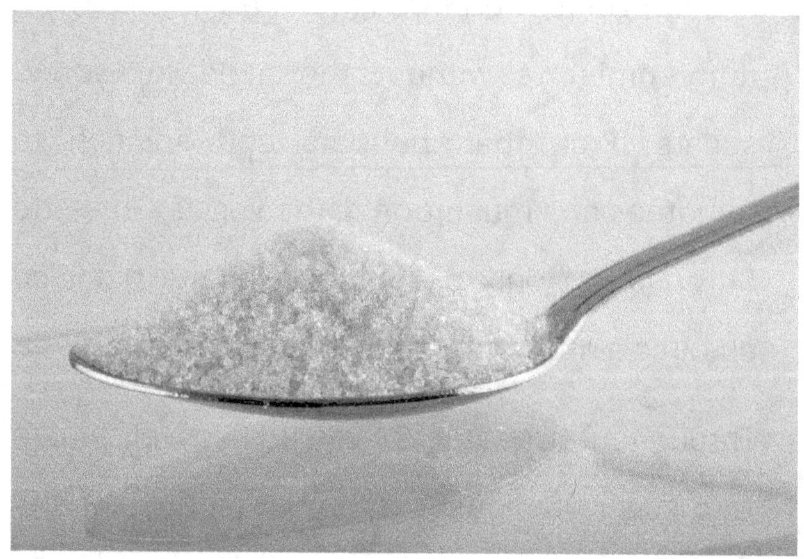

Chapter 4:

Lunchtime Favorites

As the day unfolds, Chapter 4 invites you to savor a delectable array of zero sugar lunchtime favorites. These recipes not only cater to your taste buds but also contribute to your journey of embracing a health-conscious lifestyle.

4.1 Grilled Chicken Salad with Avocado Dressing

Elevate your lunch experience with the Grilled Chicken Salad, a vibrant medley of flavors and textures. This section guides you through the art of grilling succulent chicken and assembling a nutrient-rich salad. The star of the show is the creamy Avocado Dressing, providing a luscious and satisfying alternative to sugary dressings. Packed with leafy greens, colorful vegetables, and lean protein, this salad ensures a satisfying and guilt-free midday meal.

4.2 Quinoa and Black Bean Bowl

Dive into a wholesome and protein-packed lunch with the Quinoa and Black Bean Bowl. This part of the chapter explores the versatility of quinoa, a nutrient-dense grain, and the protein richness of black beans. Enhanced with a variety of fresh vegetables, herbs, and a squeeze of lime, this bowl becomes a satisfying and flavorful option that keeps you fueled throughout the day. Say goodbye to added sugars while indulging in this savory creation.

4.3 Zucchini Noodles with Pesto

Explore the world of low-carb, zero sugar goodness with Zucchini Noodles topped with

Pesto. This section delves into the art of creating zucchini noodles, providing a healthy alternative to traditional pasta. Paired with a vibrant and herbaceous pesto sauce made from basil, pine nuts, and olive oil, this dish showcases that eliminating sugar from your meals doesn't mean sacrificing flavor. It's a lunchtime favorite that promises both satisfaction and nutritional value.

In Chapter 4, you'll discover that lunch can be a celebration of flavors, textures, and health. From the Grilled Chicken Salad with Avocado Dressing to the Quinoa and Black Bean Bowl, and the Zucchini Noodles with Pesto, each recipe invites you to savor the joys of zero sugar cooking. Welcome to a lunchtime filled with nourishing and delightful creations that not only

please your palate but also contribute to your
overall well-being.

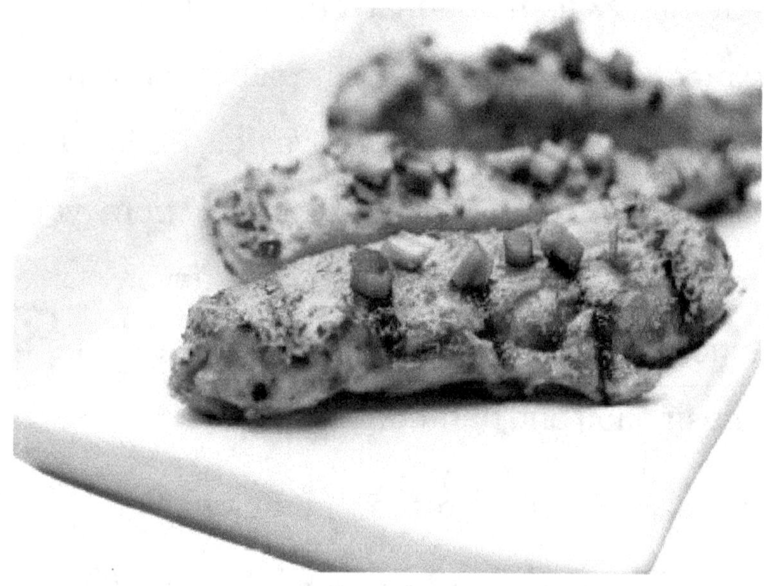

Chapter 5:

Dinner Creations

As the day concludes, Chapter 5 unveils a collection of zero sugar dinner creations that transform the evening meal into a delightful and health-conscious experience. From succulent seafood to savory stir-fries and inventive pizza alternatives, these recipes redefine dinner as a celebration of flavor and well-being.

5.1 Baked Salmon with Lemon and Herbs

Indulge in the richness of omega-3 fatty acids with the Baked Salmon featuring Lemon and Herbs. This section of the chapter guides you through the art of preparing salmon fillets seasoned with a zesty blend of lemon and aromatic herbs. The result is a mouthwatering and nutritious dish that showcases the natural flavors of the salmon without the need for added sugars. This dinner creation promises to be a culinary highlight, bringing both elegance and health to your evening meal.

5.2 Turkey and Vegetable Stir-Fry

Elevate your dinner with the savory delights of a Turkey and Vegetable Stir-Fry. This part of the chapter explores the quick and versatile world of stir-frying, combining lean turkey with an array of vibrant vegetables. The stir-fry sauce, crafted without added sugars, enhances the dish with umami flavors. It's a quick, flavorful, and nutrient-packed option for busy evenings, proving that wholesome dinners can be both convenient and delicious.

5.3 Cauliflower Pizza Crust with Veggie Toppings

Bid farewell to traditional pizza crusts laden with refined sugars and embrace the inventive Cauliflower Pizza Crust with Veggie Toppings. This section delves into the art of creating a low-carb and zero sugar pizza crust using cauliflower as the base. Topped with an assortment of colorful vegetables, this pizza not only satisfies pizza cravings but also showcases the creative possibilities of zero sugar cooking. It's a dinner creation that combines ingenuity with health-conscious choices.

In Chapter 5, dinner becomes a symphony of flavors and textures, each recipe a testament to the art of zero sugar cooking. Whether you're savoring the Baked Salmon with Lemon and Herbs, delighting in the Turkey and Vegetable

Stir-Fry, or relishing the Cauliflower Pizza Crust with Veggie Toppings, these dinner creations redefine the evening meal as a culinary journey towards health and taste. Welcome to a world where every bite is a celebration of well-being.

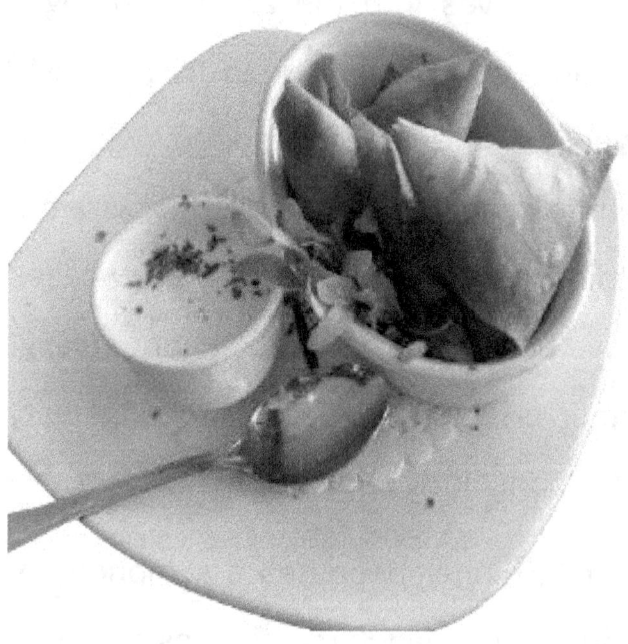

Chapter 6:

Snack Attack

As cravings strike between meals, Chapter 6 invites you to indulge in a Snack Attack that is both satisfying and health-conscious. This chapter explores a trio of snacks that redefine the art of snacking, providing a burst of flavors without compromising on your commitment to a zero sugar lifestyle.

6.1 Roasted Chickpeas

Transform humble chickpeas into a crunchy and flavorful snack with the Roasted Chickpeas recipe. This section of the chapter guides you through the process of seasoning chickpeas with an array of savory spices and roasting them to perfection. Say goodbye to sugary and processed snacks as you welcome this protein-packed, fiber-rich alternative that satiates your snack cravings while contributing to your nutritional goals.

6.2 Cheese and Nut Platter

Elevate your snacking experience with the sophistication of a Cheese and Nut Platter. This part of the chapter explores the world of artisanal cheeses paired with a variety of nuts. Rich in healthy fats and protein, this snack not only satisfies your taste buds but also keeps you satiated between meals. It's a snack attack that embraces the luxurious simplicity of quality ingredients without the need for added sugars.

6.3 Fresh Fruit Skewers

Satisfy your sweet cravings the natural way with Fresh Fruit Skewers. This section delves into the art of creating vibrant and enticing fruit skewers, combining an array of naturally sweet fruits. The result is a visually appealing and refreshing snack that celebrates the sweetness inherent in fruits without any added sugars. It's a snack attack that proves that indulgence and health-conscious choices can go hand in hand.

In Chapter 6, snacking becomes an art form, with each recipe designed to satiate your cravings while aligning with the principles of a zero sugar diet. Whether you're enjoying the crunch of Roasted Chickpeas, savoring the sophistication of a Cheese and Nut Platter, or relishing the natural sweetness of Fresh Fruit Skewers, these snacks redefine the snack attack as a journey towards mindful and flavorful indulgence. Welcome to a world where snacking is not just about filling the gap but about celebrating the art of delicious and health-conscious choices.

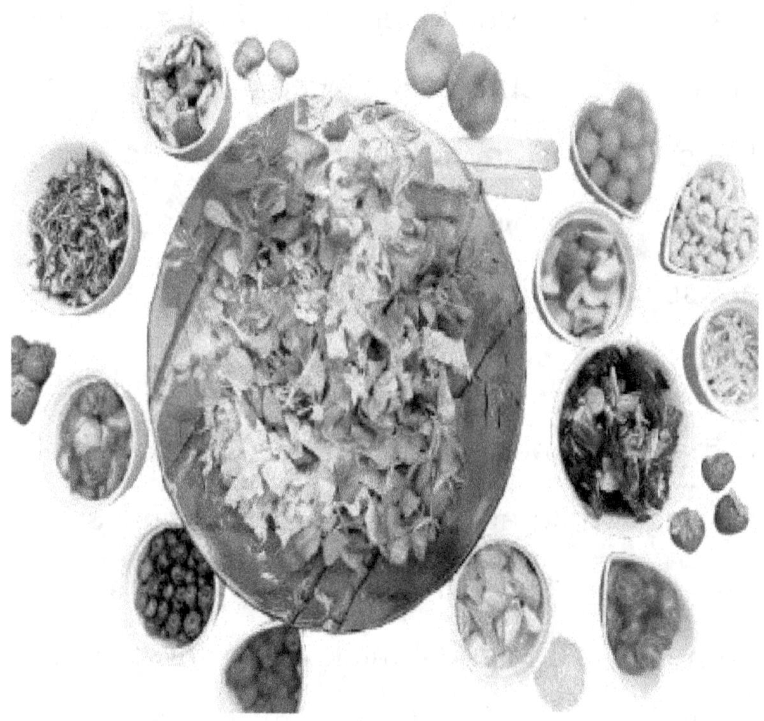

Snack Attack

How It's Prepared

When the snack cravings hit, indulge in a Snack Attack that's not only delicious but also aligns with the principles of a zero sugar lifestyle. In this section, we'll explore the step-by-step preparations for three enticing and health-conscious snacks: Roasted Chickpeas, Cheese and Nut Platter, and Fresh Fruit Skewers.

1. Roasted Chickpeas

Ingredients:

Canned chickpeas

Olive oil

Spices (paprika, cumin, garlic powder, salt, pepper)

Preparation: Preheat your oven to 400°F (200°C).Rinse and drain the canned chickpeas thoroughly.

Pat the chickpeas dry with a clean kitchen towel to remove excess moisture.

In a bowl, toss the chickpeas with olive oil, paprika, cumin, garlic powder, salt, and pepper. Ensure the chickpeas are evenly coated.

Spread the seasoned chickpeas on a baking sheet in a single layer.

Roast in the preheated oven for 25-30 minutes or until the chickpeas are golden and crispy.

Allow them to cool slightly before serving. Enjoy this crunchy, protein-packed snack!

2. Cheese and Nut Platter

Ingredients:

Assorted cheeses (cheddar, brie, gouda)

Mixed nuts (almonds, walnuts, pistachios)

Fresh or dried fruits (grapes, figs, apricots)

Preparation:

Select a variety of cheeses, ensuring a mix of textures and flavors.

Arrange the cheeses on a platter, leaving space for nuts and fruits.

Add a selection of mixed nuts to the platter, creating a visual and textural contrast.

Intersperse the cheese and nut arrangement with fresh or dried fruits for sweetness and color.

Consider adding some whole-grain crackers or slices of a baguette for a complete and satisfying snack.

Serve the Cheese and Nut Platter at room temperature, allowing the flavors to shine. Enjoy the delightful combination of textures and tastes!

3. Fresh Fruit Skewers

Ingredients:

Assorted fresh fruits (strawberries, pineapple, melon, grapes)

Wooden skewers

Preparation:

Wash and prepare the fresh fruits by cutting them into bite-sized pieces.

Thread the fruit pieces onto wooden skewers, alternating colors and textures.

Arrange the Fresh Fruit Skewers on a serving platter for a visually appealing presentation.

Optionally, drizzle with a touch of honey or a sprinkle of mint for added flavor.

Serve the skewers chilled or at room temperature for a refreshing and naturally sweet snack. Savor the goodness of nature

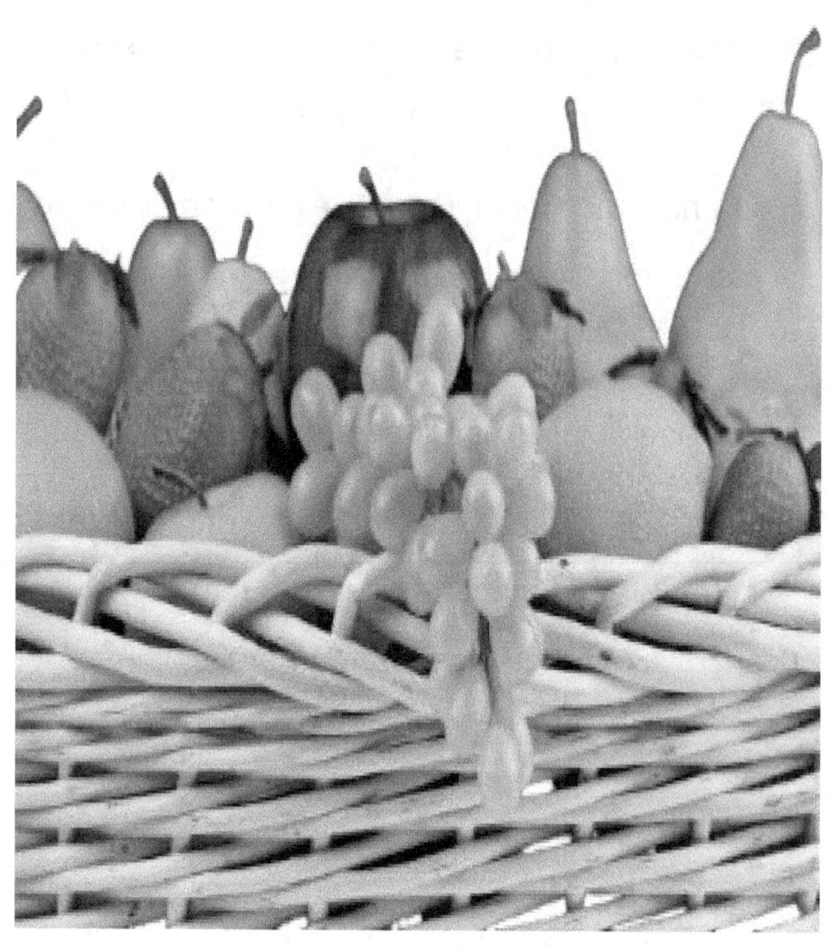

Chapter 7:

Sweet Treats without the Sugar

Satisfy your sweet tooth without compromising your commitment to a sugar-free lifestyle. Chapter 7 unveils a trio of decadent and health-conscious sweet treats: Sugar-Free Dark Chocolate Mousse, Berry Parfait, and Cinnamon Baked Apples. Dive into the world of guilt-free indulgence and discover the step-by-step preparations for these delightful desserts.

1. Sugar-Free Dark Chocolate Mousse

Ingredients:

Avocados

Unsweetened cocoa powder

Sugar-free sweetener (stevia or monk fruit)

Almond milk

Vanilla extract

Pinch of salt

Preparation:

Peel and pit the avocados, placing the flesh in a blender or food processor.

Add unsweetened cocoa powder, sugar-free sweetener, almond milk, vanilla extract, and a pinch of salt to the blender.

Blend the ingredients until smooth and creamy, adjusting sweetness to taste.

Refrigerate the mixture for at least 2 hours to allow it to set.

Serve the Sugar-Free Dark Chocolate Mousse chilled, garnished with a sprinkle of cocoa powder or fresh berries. Enjoy the rich and velvety goodness guilt-free!

2. Berry Parfait

Ingredients:

Greek yogurt

Mixed berries (strawberries, blueberries, raspberries)

Sugar-free granola

Sugar-free sweetener (optional)

Preparation:

In serving glasses or bowls, layer Greek yogurt with mixed berries.

Optionally, add a sprinkle of sugar-free sweetener to the Greek yogurt for extra sweetness.

Continue layering until the glass is almost full, finishing with a layer of berries on top.

Top the parfait with a generous amount of sugar-free granola for added crunch.

Refrigerate the Berry Parfait for at least 30 minutes before serving. Indulge in the delightful combination of creamy yogurt, fresh berries, and crunchy granola.

3. Cinnamon Baked Apples

Ingredients:

Apples

Cinnamon

Sugar-free sweetener (stevia or monk fruit)

Almond slices (optional)

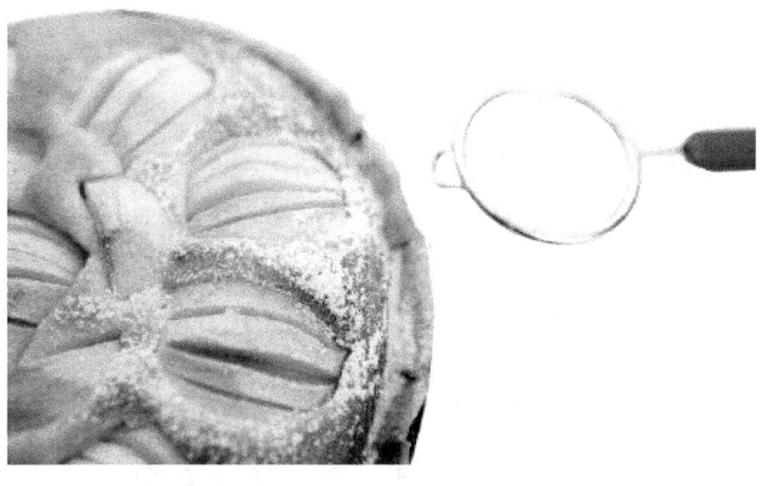

Preparation:

Preheat the oven to 375°F (190°C).

Core and slice the apples, leaving the peel on for added fiber.

In a bowl, toss the apple slices with cinnamon and sugar-free sweetener.

Arrange the coated apple slices in a baking dish.

Optionally, sprinkle almond slices on top for added texture.

Bake in the preheated oven for 25-30 minutes or until the apples are tender.

Serve the warm Cinnamon Baked Apples as a comforting and naturally sweet dessert. Enjoy the aroma of cinnamon and the natural sweetness of the apples.

Chapter 7 demonstrates that sweet treats can be both indulgent and health-conscious. Whether you're savoring the velvety texture of Sugar-Free Dark Chocolate Mousse, delighting in the layers of the Berry Parfait, or relishing the warm comfort of Cinnamon Baked Apples, each dessert is a testament to the art of creating delightful sweetness without the need for added sugars. Welcome to a world where every bite is a guilt-free celebration of flavor and well-being.with every bite!

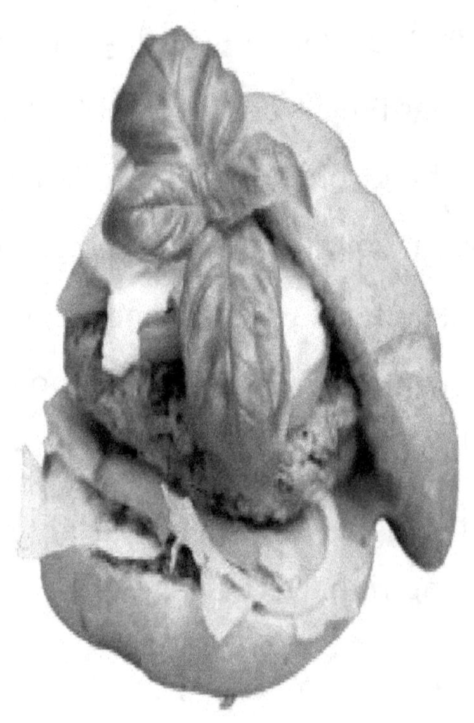

Chapter 8:

Drinks and Beverages

Quench your thirst and elevate your hydration experience with Chapter 8's collection of refreshing and health-conscious drinks and beverages. From soothing herbal teas to hydrating infused water and nutritious sugar-free smoothie recipes, this chapter is your guide to delicious and mindful sips.

1. Herbal Teas

Ingredients:

Assorted herbal tea bags (peppermint, chamomile, hibiscus, etc.)

Hot water

Optional: Fresh lemon slices, mint leaves, or a touch of honey (for sweetness)

Preparation:

Boil hot water and pour it over your chosen herbal tea bag in a cup.

Let the tea steep for the recommended time, typically 5-7 minutes.

Customize your herbal tea with fresh lemon slices, mint leaves, or a touch of honey if desired.

Experiment with different herbal tea combinations for a variety of flavors and potential health benefits.

Enjoy the soothing and aromatic experience of your personalized herbal tea.

2. Infused Water

Ingredients:

Filtered water

Assorted fruits (berries, citrus slices, cucumber)

Fresh herbs (mint, basil)

Optional: Ice cubes

Preparation:

Fill a pitcher with filtered water.

Add your choice of fruits and herbs to the water.

Refrigerate the infused water for at least 2 hours to allow the flavors to meld.

Serve the infused water over ice for a refreshing and visually appealing beverage.

Experiment with different fruit and herb combinations to find your favorite infused water blend.

3. Sugar-Free Smoothie Recipes

Ingredients:

Assorted fruits (berries, banana, mango, etc.)

Leafy greens (spinach, kale)

Greek yogurt or dairy-free alternative

Unsweetened almond milk or coconut water

Ice cubes

Preparation:

In a blender, combine your chosen fruits, leafy greens, Greek yogurt, and a liquid base.

Add ice cubes for a chilled and thicker consistency.

Blend until smooth, adjusting the liquid as needed for the desired thickness.

Customize your sugar-free smoothie with additional ingredients like chia seeds or a sprinkle of cinnamon.

Pour the smoothie into a glass and enjoy this nutrient-packed and naturally sweet beverage.

In Chapter 8, your drink choices become a delightful exploration of flavors, hydration, and health-conscious options. Whether you're sipping on the soothing notes of Herbal Teas, hydrating with the vibrant Infused Water, or enjoying the nutrition-packed goodness of Sugar-Free Smoothie Recipes, each beverage is a celebration of mindful and flavorful sips. Welcome to a world where your drink choices contribute not only to your hydration but also to your overall well-being.

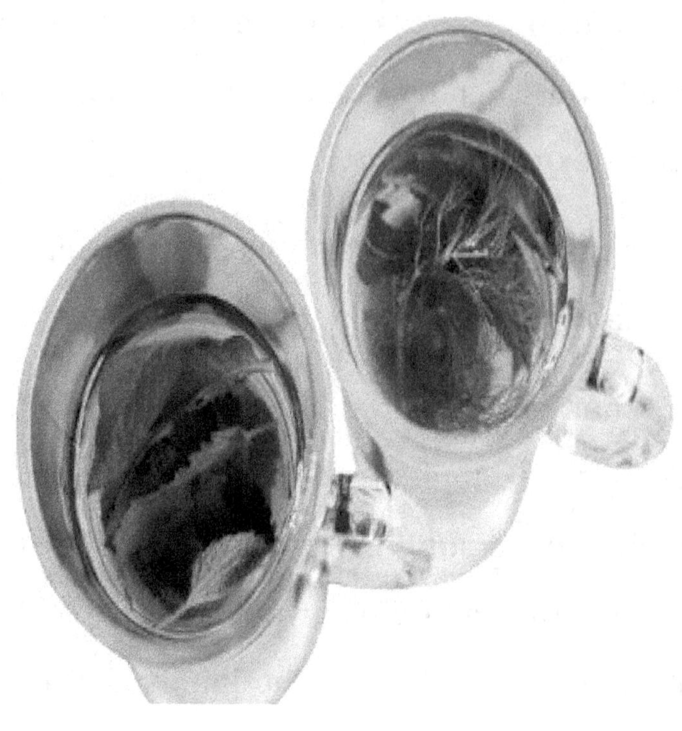

Chapter 9: Tips for Dining Out

Navigating the world of dining out while adhering to a zero sugar lifestyle can present challenges, but with strategic planning and informed choices, you can still enjoy meals at restaurants and navigate social gatherings seamlessly. Chapter 9 provides valuable insights and practical tips to make dining out a positive and health-conscious experience.

1. Making Smart Choices at Restaurants

Understanding Menus:

Scan for Sugar-Free Options: Look for dishes labeled as sugar-free, low-carb, or keto-friendly.

Choose Grilled Over Fried: Opt for grilled or baked dishes rather than fried options to reduce hidden sugars.

Customize Your Order: Don't hesitate to ask for modifications, such as no added sauces, dressings on the side, or substitutions for starchy sides.

Smart Choices by Cuisine:

Asian Cuisine: Lean towards stir-fries with vegetables and protein, avoiding sweet sauces.

Italian Cuisine: Opt for grilled proteins, salads, and dishes with tomato-based sauces, avoiding pasta and creamy sauces.

Mexican Cuisine: Choose fajitas with lean protein, skip the tortillas, and focus on salsa, guacamole, and veggies.

Managing Portions:

Share or Half Portions: Consider sharing dishes or asking for half portions to control portion sizes.

Start with a Salad: Begin your meal with a salad to help control hunger and potentially reduce overall calorie intake.

2. Handling Social Gatherings

Communicating Dietary Needs:

Inform Hosts in Advance: If possible, let hosts know about your dietary preferences or restrictions ahead of time.

Ask for Ingredient Lists: If uncertain about ingredients, politely ask for details to make informed choices.

Navigating Buffets and Potlucks:

Survey the Options: Take a quick overview of the buffet or potluck offerings before serving yourself.

Focus on Protein and Veggies: Prioritize protein-rich and vegetable-based dishes to avoid excessive carbs and sugars.

Coping with Peer Pressure:

Be Confident in Your Choices: Politely decline offers of foods that don't align with your dietary goals, and confidently make choices that support your well-being.

Suggest Alternatives: If possible, suggest alternative venues or contribute a dish to social gatherings to ensure there are options aligned with your preferences.

Dining out and socializing should be enjoyable experiences, and with these practical tips, you can navigate restaurant menus and gatherings with confidence. Chapter 9 empowers you to make informed choices, communicate effectively, and maintain your commitment to a zero sugar lifestyle while still enjoying the pleasures of dining out and socializing with friends and family.

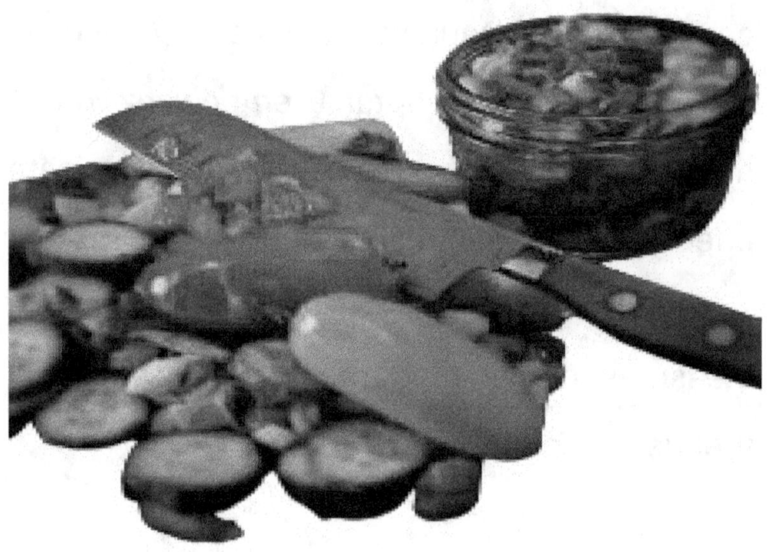

Chapter 10:

Meal Planning and Prepping

Efficient meal planning and preparation are integral to maintaining a zero sugar lifestyle. Chapter 10 introduces you to the art of crafting weekly meal plans, adopting batch cooking strategies for convenience, and smart shopping practices to ensure your kitchen is stocked with zero sugar essentials.

1. Weekly Meal Plans

Strategizing Your Week:

Designate Planning Time: Dedicate a specific time each week to plan your meals and snacks.

Balance Macronutrients: Ensure your meals include a balance of lean proteins, healthy fats, and low-carb vegetables to support your nutritional goals.

Incorporate Variety: Keep your palate engaged by including a variety of flavors, textures, and cuisines throughout the week.

Meal Prep Checklist:

Prepare a Shopping List: Based on your planned meals, create a comprehensive shopping list to streamline grocery trips.

Chop and Portion Ingredients: Spend some time washing, chopping, and portioning vegetables, fruits, and proteins for easy access during the week.

Precook Staples: Cook grains, proteins, and other staples in advance to reduce the time required for meal assembly on busy days.

2. Batch Cooking for Convenience

Time-Saving Benefits:

Efficient Use of Time: Batch cooking allows you to prepare larger quantities of food at once, minimizing daily cooking efforts.

Freezer-Friendly Options: Many dishes can be frozen in individual portions for future use, providing a convenient solution for busy days.

Batch Cooking Tips:

Choose Versatile Ingredients: Opt for ingredients that can be used in multiple dishes throughout the week.

Utilize Slow Cookers and Instant Pots: These appliances are excellent for batch cooking and require minimal hands-on time.

Label and Date Portions: Properly label and date your batch-cooked portions for easy identification in the freezer.

3. Smart Shopping for Zero Sugar

Planning Before Shopping:

Create a Shopping List: Stick to your planned meals and ingredients to avoid impulse purchases.

Shop with Purpose: Focus on the perimeter of the grocery store, where fresh produce, proteins, and dairy are typically located.

Navigating the Aisles:

Read Labels Carefully: Scrutinize food labels to identify hidden sugars and choose products with minimal processing.

Choose Whole Foods: for whole, unprocessed foods to ensure you have control over the ingredients in your meals.

Stocking Up on Staples:

Zero Sugar Pantry Essentials: Keep your pantry stocked with essentials like herbs, spices, sugar alternatives, and low-carb flours to facilitate zero sugar cooking.

Purchase in Bulk: Buy non-perishable items in bulk to save money and reduce the frequency of shopping trips.

Chapter 10 empowers you to take control of your meal planning and preparation, making the journey towards a zero sugar lifestyle more achievable and sustainable. By adopting weekly meal plans, embracing batch cooking for convenience, and adopting smart shopping practices, you set the foundation for success in maintaining a health-conscious and flavorful approach to your meals.

CONCLUSION:

Nourishing a Zero Sugar Lifestyle

In the culinary journey of "Nourishing a Zero Sugar Lifestyle," each chapter unfolds as a roadmap, guiding you through the intricacies of adopting a health-conscious, flavorful, and sustainable approach to nutrition. As we conclude this comprehensive guide, let's reflect on the valuable insights and practical strategies gleaned from the diverse chapters that have paved the way for your transformative journey.

Chapter 1 to 3: Foundation for Transformation

In the initial chapters, we laid the groundwork for a zero sugar lifestyle. Understanding the impact of sugars on health, delving into the benefits of a zero sugar diet for managing diabetes, and establishing the key principles and guidelines provided the foundation for the transformative journey that followed.

Chapter 4 to 6: Crafting Culinary Delights

From breakfast to dinner and snack times in between, Chapters 4 to 6 celebrated the art of crafting zero sugar culinary delights. Each recipe unveiled in these chapters beckons you to explore the richness of flavors while maintaining a commitment to health-conscious choices. Whether savoring Veggie Omelette Surprises or enjoying the crunch of Roasted Chickpeas, these creations prove that nourishing meals can be both a delight to the palate and a boon to well-being.

Chapter 7 to 9: Indulging in Sweet Treats, Smart Dining, and Beverage Mastery

In the pursuit of a sugar-free sweet tooth fix, Chapter 7 presented a trio of desserts that showcase indulgence without compromise. Meanwhile, Chapter 8 took you on a journey through refreshing drinks and beverages, ensuring your hydration aligns with your health goals. Chapter 9 equipped you with practical tips for dining out, empowering you to make informed choices and gracefully navigate social gatherings while staying true to your zero sugar commitment.

Chapter 10: Mastering Meal Planning and Preparation

The concluding chapter encapsulates the essence of sustainable change. By providing guidance on crafting weekly meal plans, embracing the efficiency of batch cooking, and adopting smart shopping practices, you are now equipped with the tools to seamlessly integrate a zero sugar lifestyle into your routine. The art of meal planning and preparation becomes not just a necessity but a source of empowerment, allowing you to take control of your nutrition and well-being.

In closing, "Nourishing a Zero Sugar Lifestyle" is more than a culinary guide; it's a holistic approach to health and flavor. It is a journey that invites you to savor the joys of mindful eating, embrace the art of crafting nutritious and delicious meals, and find empowerment in making informed choices for a life nourished by health and well-being. May this guide be a steadfast companion in your ongoing quest for a vibrant, zero sugar lifestyle.